Leila TRIKI
Sana SELLAMI

Neurophysiological characterization of chemically induced neuropathies

Leila TRIKI
Sana SELLAMI

Neurophysiological characterization of chemically induced neuropathies

: case-control study

ScienciaScripts

Cover image: www.ingimage.com

This book is a translation from the original published under ISBN 978-620-3-44523-7.

Publisher:
Sciencia Scripts
is a trademark of
Dodo Books Indian Ocean Ltd. and OmniScriptum S.R.L publishing group

120 High Road, East Finchley, London, N2 9ED, United Kingdom
Str. Armeneasca 28/1, office 1, Chisinau MD-2012, Republic of Moldova, Europe
Printed at: see last page
ISBN: 978-620-5-89997-7

Plan

Introduction

Chemo-induced peripheral neuropathy (CIPN) is a frequent complication (1). These chemotherapies for which patients present symptoms in the short term are most often platinum derivatives (PD) and Taxanes. The neurotoxicity of these molecules has long been reported (1-3). Their indications are often similar (4, 5). However, it would appear that their neurotoxic effects do not have the same weight chronologically (6). In fact, the side effects of Taxanes would be earlier than those of PDs (6). In the face of this neuropathic damage, patients would first present positive sensory symptoms including pain (dysesthesia, allodynia, hyperpathy), tingling (paresthesias), and/or numbness typically localized in the hands and feet. Motor symptoms are more common than autonomic symptoms and occur with Taxanes but are rare with PDs since they must cross the blood-brain barrier to affect the anterior horn cells. Motor symptoms would often present as distal or general weakness, muscle cramps, or instability on walking.

Autonomic symptoms may present as constipation or diarrhea, swallowing abnormalities, dizziness and/or vertigo with changes in position, which may be associated with loss of temperature or vibration sensation, or orthostatic hypotension (7).

Proprioceptive ataxia could occur and would be explained by damage to peripheral proprioceptive pathways (large diameter myelinated sensory fibers, spinal ganglion) or central ones (posterior cords of the spinal cord and relays) causing a deficit in deep sensibility (vibrations, sense of position and movement) responsible for ataxia and sometimes tremor.

The diagnosis of CINP is usually made on clinical grounds, but electrophysiology can help confirm the diagnosis of CINP and exclude other etiologies of neuropathic signs and symptoms (7). Electroneuromyographic examination (ENMG) is not included in the guidelines in routine practice.

It is an examination that allows exploration of the large nerve fibers of the nerve trunks and evaluation of the degree of their damage (8-10). Indeed, this examination makes it possible to quantify the degree of axonal loss in the large-caliber sensitive and motor fibers, and whether or not this loss is associated with a decrease in nerve conduction velocities. It allows to characterize the truncal nerve damage, to localize it and to specify if this damage is length-dependent or not (1, 10, 11). Toxic neuropathies are mostly length-dependent (1), however, sensory neuronopathies have been described (12) and are often more difficult to diagnose. Involvement of the autonomic nervous system has also been described, but this would be rarer, particularly with PD and Taxanes (1).

ENMG is often performed without delay at the onset of symptoms (within the first week) in our department in order toidentify distal peripheral nerve damage of the large nerve fibers, which would guide subsequent management in order to continue or stop treatment. The diagnosis of neuropathy can only be retained if it is supported by conduction abnormalities, mainly sensory, recorded on the ENMG in favor of a truncal nerve damage. The purpose of this study would be to clarify the value of ENMG in the diagnosis of NPCI and whether it allows objective characterization of neuropathies secondary to Taxanes and PD.

Physiopathology

Taxanes :

a) Definition:

The name taxanes comes from the Latin term Taxus sp found in these ornamental plants, which have long been known to be toxic. Paclitaxel (PCTX) was the first drug in this group isolated from the stem bark of the Pacific yew in 1960, although it was not approved for use in ovarian cancer until 1994 (13). Docetaxel (DCTX) is a semi-synthetic derivative of paclitaxel. Both drugs are highly insoluble; they require different solvents, which frequently induce allergic reactions. Thus, research on a new generation of taxanes is aimed at obtaining molecules with better therapeutic and toxic profiles and higher solubility (14).

B) Mechanism of action:

Taxanes block cell division by disrupting the spindle through an impact on microtubules. Microtubules play an essential role at every stage of the cell cycle from the DNA synthesis phase to cell division. They are essential components of the mitotic spindle that guide the separation of genetic material from the mother cell to the two daughter cells. They are also involved in the maintenance of the cytoskeleton.

The taxanes are chemically very similar and therefore have a similar, dose-dependent mechanism of action. At high concentrations, PCTX binds to the βtubulin subunit, which promotes the assembly of tubulin-enhancing microtubule polymerization. Impaired mitotic spindle formation prevents normal mitosis and cells undergo apoptosis. On the other hand, low concentrations of PCTX do not increase microtubule polymerization, but act as microtubule stabilizing agents, blocking depolymerization, so that anaphase cannot be reached and apoptosis mechanisms are activated (15).

Although chemically quite similar, DCTX and PCTX show some differences in mechanism of action. The tubulin polymers generated by DCTX are structured differently than those of PCTX, and DCTX does not alter the number of protofilaments in microtubules (16).

Most previous studies have shown that the incidence of PCTX-induced neuropathy is higher than that of DCTX (17, 18), although there is some controversy because it is not always observed (14). Taxane-induced neuropathy primarily affects small diameter sensory fibers, inducing impaired proprioception and paresthesias, dysesthesias, and numbness in a distal glove distribution.

Accordingly, PCTX treatment has been associated with a reduction in sensory nerve action potential and a reduction in sensitive nerve conduction velocity (19). Motor and autonomic dysfunctions are less likely to occur.

Axons of sensory neurons are highly active in the retrograde and anterograde transport of different molecules, which is necessary for their survival and is dependent on microtubules (20). Several studies have pointed out that taxane-induced alterations in microtubule structure could impair axonal transport and, consequently, cause degeneration of distal nerve segments (21).

Studies have observed PCTX-induced changes in acetylated tubulin, but tubulin expression rapidly returns to control levels after drug treatment is discontinued, whereas morphological effects persist long after treatment (22).

Interestingly, although PCTX does not cause direct mitochondrial DNA damage, mitochondria have been suggested as potential mediators of PCTX toxicity, as swollen and vacuolated mitochondria have been observed in both myelinated and unmyelinated sensory nerves, such that the authors conclude that mitochondrial alterations contribute to PCTX-induced pain rather than axonal microtubule dysfunction (23).

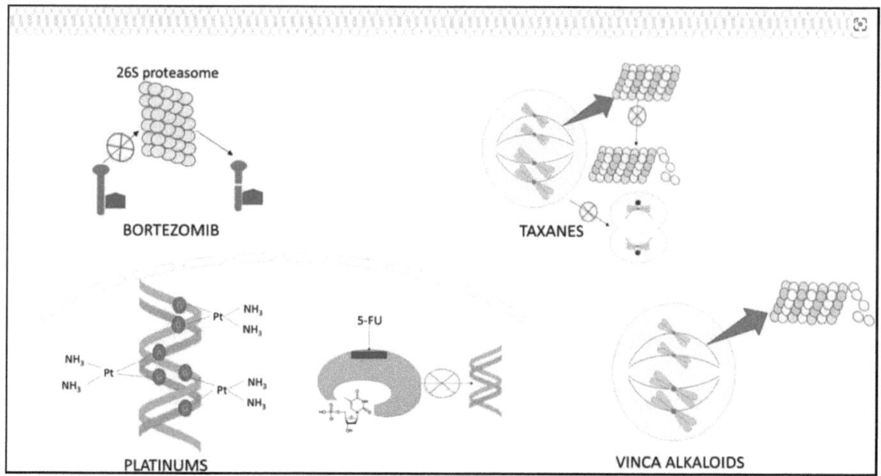

Figure: Schematic representation of the mechanisms of action of the main antitumor drugs responsible for direct neurotoxicity and peripheral neuropathy.

1) Bortezomib inhibits the 26S proteasome.

2) Taxanes stabilize tubulin proteins, so anaphase cannot be reached.

3) Vinca alkaloids destabilize microtubules, so the mitotic spindle cannot be formed.

4) Platinum-based compounds form intrastrand and cross-strand bonds.

5) 5- Fluorouracil (5-FU) binds to thymidylate synthase (TS). (24)

Platinum derivatives :

A) Definition:

The first antitumor agent in this group was cisplatin, patented in 1978 for the treatment of various types of solid tumors. However, because of its side effects and the development of cellular resistance, carboplatin (a second-generation platinum agent) and oxaliplatin (a third-generation platinum agent) are now the most frequently used in the clinic (25).

Mode of administration:

Platinum agents are administered intravenously and enter the cell by passive diffusion, but also by active transport (26). Once entered, all platinum agents become aquated and, although they interact with ribonucleic acid (RNA) and proteins, the primary target is deoxynucleic acid (DNA). All platinum agents preferentially bind to guanosine and adenosine, to form intrastrand and interstrand cross-links (27).

Mechanism of Action:

Platinum salts are alkylating agents, capable of binding to DNA by attaching an alkyl group (CnH2n+1) to a guanine base at the nitrogen position 7 of the purine ring. This forms abnormal bridges between the two strands of DNA1. The DNA-platinum complex, called an adduct, inhibits DNA replication by blocking the progression of replication enzymes along the molecule. Cytotoxicity is thus dependent on the amount of platinum bound to the DNA.

A) Mechanism of neurotoxicity:

The primary mechanism by which platinum compounds induce neuropathy is primarily due to the DNA adducts they form in the nucleus of neurons. Some of these adducts are less efficiently repaired by the nucleotide excision repair (NER) pathway, so that platinum-DNA adducts that are not removed by NER do not allow for proper ribosomal RNA transcription. DRG neurons are highly metabolic cells and thus the absence of dense physiological ribosomal RNA synthesis can be lethal to this cell type (28).

Platinum compounds also have the ability to bind to mitochondrial DNA (mtDNA), which cannot be repaired because there is no DNA repair system in mitochondria, thereby increasing the amount of reactive oxygen species (ROS) and oxidative stress (29).

Mitochondria and the endoplasmic reticulum are internal stores for Ca2+; when damaged, intracellular Ca2+ levels are increased, resulting in altered neuronal excitability and activation

of calpain causing axonal degeneration (30).
Recently, the role of the gut microbiota has been implicated in the development of oxaliplatin-induced peripheral sensory neuropathy. Chronic administration of oxaliplatin did not induce mechanical hypersensitivity in mice or spontaneous pain behavior in antibiotic-pretreated rats or germ-free mice, whereas neuropathy occurred in control animals (31).

The authors found that the microbiota influenced the development of oxaliplatin-induced mechanical hypersensitivity through a lipopolysaccharide (LPS)-TLR4 pathway and that TLR4 expression on hematopoietic cells appears to be at least partially responsible for this effect (31).

- Cisplatin:

1/ Nature, indication and mechanism of action of the drug :

Cisplatinum or cis-dichlorodiamminoplatinum (DDP) is a cytotoxic anticancer drug that has been used since 1972 in the United States and since 1979 in France. It is a heavy metal complex with a central platinum atom. It is indicated for ovarian, testicular, bladder, head and neck, endometrial, small cell bronchial cancers and solid tumors in children. It acts by inhibiting DNA synthesis through the formation of chromosomal intra- and inter-strand bonds.

2/ Clinical aspects:

The clinical picture is stereotyped, reflecting the almost exclusive involvement of the large sensory fibers. Initially, patients complain of paresthesias and numbness of the extremities of the limbs before reaching the lower limbs, which can also be rapidly painful. Then appear balance disorders related to an ataxia, sometimes very disabling. Pallesthesia is precociously altered, as well as arthrokinetic and tactile sensitivities.

In contrast, thermoalgesic sensitivity is relatively preserved. Reflexes are diminished or abolished, but muscle strength is well preserved with rare exceptions (32). Associated cochlear toxicity is common. A hermits sign is sometimes present. Neuropathy may appear after cessation of treatment or continue to progress for several months after cessation of cisplatin treatment, a freewheeling phenomenon.

4/ Electrophysiological study:

In most cases, EMG and motor conduction velocities are normal. Increased latencies and decreased amplitude of sensory potentials are in favor of axonal degeneration. In a few cases, disturbances of cortical sensory evoked potentials are more important than the peripheral involvement would suggest a centroperipheral axonopathy with posterior cord degeneration. In more advanced forms, motor conduction velocities may be reduced and distal motor potentials may be of reduced amplitude. Simultaneous involvement of sensory potentials in the upper and lower limbs is also a characteristic feature, suggesting an initial lesion of the posterior spinal ganglion. The early alteration of the H reflex of the soleus muscle is sometimes contrasted with the relative preservation of the amplitudes of the distal sensory potentials, notably of the sural nerve, which would also be suggestive of an initial damage to the posterior spinal ganglion. Involvement of the autonomic nervous system is rare and poorly documented (33).

3/ Evolution:

Cisplatin-induced neuropathy is reversible, but recovery may be long, requiring a few months to more than a year. Residual manifestations, especially sensory ones, may persist for many years after the initial high-dose treatment has been stopped.

- Carboplatin:

Carboplatin is very similar to cisplatin but has less neurotoxicity at conventional doses. It is used in resistant ovarian cancers, often in combination with paclitaxel. Neuropathy is usually moderate and affects only 6% of treated patients. Severe forms of neuropathy occur only at very high doses (34).

- Oxaliplatin:

It is mainly used in colorectal cancer with metastasis.

It acts by cross-linking with DNA and by blocking the synthesis of the DNA. Oxaliplatin induces neuropathy by a novel mechanism by interfering with axonal ionic conductance and thus altering nerve excitability. Oxaliplatin-induced neuropathy may be chronic, in all respects similar to that induced by cisplatin, or more rarely acute, triggered by cold, purely sensitive and rapidly reversible (35).

Drug-induced toxic neuropathies:

Although not common, toxic neuropathies due to medication deserve to be known and identified. Numerous trials are currently underway on substances likely to protect the patient against the neurotoxicity of the product administered. Some of them are very promising and the development of research in this direction also seems to be rich in possibilities for the understanding and treatment of neuropathies outside of any toxic drug intake. Other products are toxic in a random way and affect very few patients. It is possible that predisposing factors are involved. It is also necessary to use certain toxic drugs only after having eliminated a pre-existing neuropathy, such as a hereditary neuropathy which could present a rapid and severe aggravation.

Importantly, compared to the central nervous system (CNS), the peripheral nervous system (PNS) is not protected by a structure similar to the blood-brain barrier (BBB), and therefore faces direct toxicity.

The effects of antineoplastic drugs on peripheral neurons are considerable, but also indirect, contributing effects, mainly due to inflammatory reactions, leading to the development of chemotherapy-induced peripheral neuropathy (CIPN)

NPIC is a widespread, severe, dose-limiting toxicity, resulting in dose interruptions and subtherapeutic administration (23). Acute symptoms of CIPN occur within hours and days of drug infusion, and persistent symptoms occur in approximately 68% of patients 1 month after completion of chemotherapy (36).

Neuropathic pain is characterized by the presence of allodynia and hyperalgesia due to the decreased sensitivity threshold for non-harmful and harmful stimuli, respectively. Remarkably, spontaneous pain may also be present in some patients. Similarly, peripheral motor nerves may be affected by some drugs, leading to motor deficits (37).

Basic agents (oxaliplatin, cisplatin, carboplatin), taxanes (paclitaxel, docetaxel), vinca alkaloids (vincristine, vinblastine), proteasome inhibitors and thalidomide analogues can cause direct neurotoxicity and NPIC (37).

Knowing how these agents interact with the nervous system is crucial for the development of drugs that can protect against peripheral neuropathy.

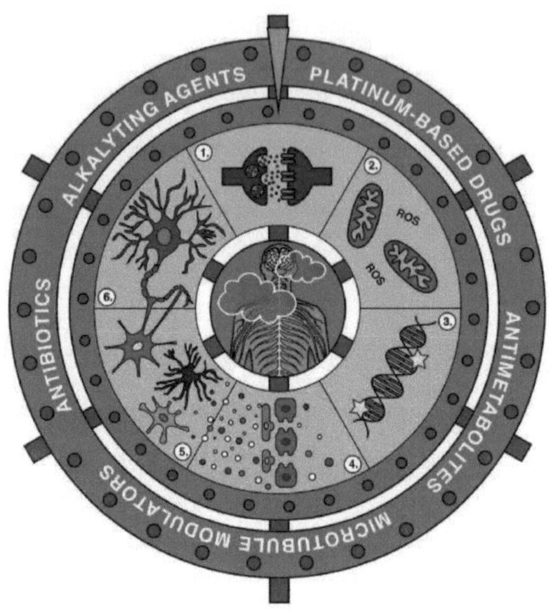

Figure 1: chemically induced neuropathy: (24)

1. secretion of down-regulated neurotransmitters,
2. overproduction of reactive oxygen species,
3. genetic alterations,
4. neuroinflammation and blood-brain barrier degradation,
5. reduction of gliogenesis and hyperactivation of microglia and astrocytes,
6. alteration of neurogenesis and the dynamic neural network, this will lead to the development of neural dysfunctions (neuropathic pain, cognitive deficits) in the majority of cancer patients.

Material and methods

This is a retrospective analytical case-control study. We were interested in studying the files of patients referred from the carcinology department for exploration by an ENMG between January 2013 and December 2020 for suspicion of NPCI. NPCI was evoked in front of:

- A motor or sensory deficit of radicular or truncal topography systematized to one (or more) roots or nerve trunks
- A decrease or abolition of the tendon reflexes which is not specific because it is also the case in the initial phase called "flaccid" central motor deficit
- Distal lower limb involvement without bladder-sphincter disorders (38).

These symptoms must have appeared after the initiation of chemotherapy (1).

41 files were collected. These records were to contain:

- All data related to the patient's clinical history: anthropometric data (age, sex,), personal history and carcinoma pathology for which the patient is being treated
- His ongoing chemotherapy treatment,
- The type of symptom presented: paresthesias
- Data from the clinician's examination: when mentioned in the liaison letter, it would specify the neurological examination performed: the search for superficial sensitivity impairment

and deep, the search for a motor deficit, the search for a cerebellar syndrome and the result of the osteotendinous reflexes. The clinician would associate a clinical grade with NPCI according to the criteria in the attached table:

Table I: Clinical assessment according to (39, 40)

	WHO	NCI	ECOG
GRADE 1	Paresthesias and/or decreased tendon reflexes	Asymptomatic, loss of tendon reflexes or paresthesias	Mild paresthesias, loss of osteotendinous reflex, subjective weakness, no signs objectives found
GRADE 2	Severe paresthesias and/or mild weakness	Moderate sensory and motor symptoms	Mild to moderate objectified sensory loss or moderate paresthesias, mild objectified weakness without impairment of function
GRADE3	Intolerable paresthesias and/or marked motor loss	Severe sensory and motor symptoms limiting self-maintenance, assistance is required	Severe sensory loss or paresthesias interfering with function, objectified weakness with impaired function
GRADE	Paralysis	Consequences life, intervention urgent indicated	Paralysis

WHO: WORLD HEALTH ORAGNISATION , NCI: NATIONAL CANCER INSTITUTE, ECOG: EASTERN COOPERATIVE ONCOLOGY GROUP

- Data collected by the ENMG examination: The nerve conduction study (or stimulus-detection) for peripheral neuropathy should include the study of sensitive nerve conduction (sensitive amplitude (μV), distal sensitive latency (ms), and sensitive conduction velocity (m/s)) and the study of motor nerve conduction (motor amplitude (μV), distal motor latency (ms) and motor conduction velocity between 2 stimulation points of the same nerve trunk (m/s) of the same nerve and the latency of the F wave (for the study of proximal conduction)). In the context of the exploration of a CINP, the examination most often includes: the study of the nerve conduction of the sural nerve, the study of the nerve conduction of the musculocutaneous nerve, the study of the motor conduction of the common fibular nerve (SPE) and the study of the motor conduction of the tibial nerve (SPI) for the lower limbs. The examination of the lower limbs is essential, especially when the diagnosis of length-dependent polyneuropathy is evoked. The examination of the upper limbs cannot be excluded but would most often be performed when the examination of the lower limbs is pathological, when the diagnosis of neuronopathy is suspected or when the patient presents signs of call (paresthesias of the hands, motor deficit. . .) inciting the realization of a study of the nerve conduction of the upper limbs, which was not studied here because of the reduced number of patients for whom the examination of the upper limbs was carried out

- The neurophysiologist's conclusion: it will specify that it is a sensitive axonal neuropathy (if the sensitive amplitude of the sural nerve is < 20 μV associated with a sensitive amplitude of the musculocutaneous nerve < 15 μV) and motor (if the motor amplitude of the SPE nerve is < 4 μV and of the SPI nerve is < 4 μV) or demyelinating neuropathy (if distal motor latencies are prolonged, conduction velocities are slowed, F-wave latencies are prolonged, if conduction block or temporal dispersion is present or if the duration of the distal potential is prolonged), however this last involvement is not frequent in the context of a NPCI This conclusion will also specify that this involvement is length-dependent (noting the symmetrical distal involvement mainly affecting the lower limbs, particularly on the sensory level, with possible involvement of the upper limbs). A multiple mononeuritis or a sensory neuronopathy can be evoked in the presence of

a multifocal, asymmetric involvement for 2 limbs. To facilitate the diagnosis of sensory neuronopathies, Camdessanché et *al.* developed a clinical and electrical score (41).

Table II: Clinical and electroneuromyographic criteria for sensory neuropathy (26)

Possible neuropathy if total score > 6.5	**yes**	**Points**
Ataxia		+ 3,1
Asymmetrical symptoms		1,7
Sensory abnormalities not only in the lower limbs		+ 2,0
At least one non-recordable sensory nerve or 3 sensory nerves with sensory action potential < 30% of the lower limit of normal in the upper limbs		+ 2,8
Less than 2 abnormal motor nerves in the lower limbs		+ 3,1
Total		

The method of carrying out the ENMG is described in the appendix (see appendix).

Included in the study:

Patients with neoplastic pathologies undergoing chemotherapy with DP and Taxanes (molecules whose neurotoxicity is well known) for the patient groups. The group of control patients was selected from patients also undergoing chemotherapy but whose neurotoxicity is either absent or rarely reported. These patients were referred to the Functional Investigation Department for an ENMG following the appearance of paresthesias of the lower limbs or of the 4 limbs. Those for whom the ENMG was performed either for the lower limbs only or for all 4 limbs were included. A group of patients referred to us for radicular involvement was also included as a control group.

Excluded from the study:

Patients excluded from this study are those:

- who had been referred for a pre-chemotherapy assessment N=3
- whose type of chemotherapy was not specified N=2 .
- whose chemotherapy discontinuation is distant N=1.
- who did not have a lower limb ENMG N=1.
- with a history of diabetes and had experienced paresthesias prior to initiation of chemotherapy N=1
- Patients with neoplasia inducing paraneoplastic polyneuropathy were excluded from the study in case the diagnosis of polyneuropathy was retained, they were not excluded in the opposite case (Paraneoplastic neuropathies are represented in a table in the appendix) (41, 42) N=2.
- treated with PD and Taxanes N=2.

<u>4 groups of patients were individualized:</u>

Group G1: Patients who were treated with PDs.

Group G2: patients who were treated with Taxanes.

Group G3: patients who have been treated with other molecules with low nerve toxicity (which do not induce or weakly induce polyneuropathy) and who have been referred for ENMG (treatment: LV5-FU2, FUN (5FU-Vinorelbine (association with polyneuropathy is described but rare, autonomic nervous system related disorders would take precedence (6)), LV5-FU2-Deticene, 5FU-Folinic acid-Compto, Methotrexate and 5FU-Folinic acid)

Group G4: patients with neuralgia symptoms (control group) who were referred to us for the exploration of L5 lumbosciatica in search of radicular damage. These are patients who may have motor conduction abnormalities in the lower limbs but without any impact on the sensitive conduction of these same limbs. These are patients who were selected according to an age match and without a history of a general pathology that could cause polyneuropathy.

The data relating to the patients were entered into an SPSS 20 file from the files of the Functional Explorations Service of Sfax. The data were found either in the liaison letter to the service or on the form on which the interrogation and the examination performed on the patient were specified. The parameters of the nerve conduction were also present in the patient's file. Statistical analysis was performed using Fisher's exact test for qualitative variables with sample (n> 5). The number of samples was doubled for the nerve conduction parameters (bilaterality of the examination), and in this case the Kruskall-Wallis test was used for the comparison of means between samples (n>10). The relationship is said to be significant when $p \leq 0.05$. The Dunn-Bonferroni post hoc test was used to specify the correlation between groups.

Results

A total of 29 chemotherapy patients were included (G1: N=17; G2: N= 6; G3: N= 6), with a sex ratio of 9/20=0.45. Patients were matched for age. Table 1 reports the anthropometric and clinical characteristics of the chemotherapy groups studied. Table 2 specifies the neoplastic pathologies for which these patients were managed.

Table III: *Anthropometric and clinical characteristics of the study population*

	G1 Platinum derivatives N=17	*G2 Taxanes N= 6*	*G3 low toxicity N= 6*	*G4 controls N=8*	*p=*
Type					
M/F	9/8	0/6	0/6	3/5	
Age	62 [34;80]*	67[47;74]*	64[48;71]*	50,5[45 ; 68]*	0,071**
Symptoms					
MI paresthesias	9	2	3		
MS paresthesias	0	0	1		
Paresthesias 4M	8	4	2		
Number of treatments	2 [1ère cure], 3 [3ème cure], 2[4ème cure], 1[5ème cure], 2[6ème cure], 1[11ème cure], 1[12ème cure], 3 : 2 since one year and 1 since 7 months. Information missing for 2.	3[1ère cure], 1[3ème cure], Information missing for 2.	1[1ère cure], 2[2ème cure], 1[5ème cure], Information missing for 2.	No cure	
Diagnosis of : olyneuropathies	5	4	0	0	0,04°°

Mononeuropathies	0	0	0	0
Neuronopathies	0	0	0	0
Demyelinating neuropathy	0	0	0	0

** median [min ;max] ; **independent samples median test ; °Fisher's exact test*

Table IV: Neoplasia in the patients studied

Type of chemotherapy used *Neoplasia*	G1 :Platinum derivatives	G2 : Taxane	G3: at low toxicity
Neuroendocrine tumor	2	0	1
Breast carcinoma	0	3	0
ADK rectum	2	0	1
CE floor of the mouth	1	0	0
ADK ovary	1	3	0
ADK sigmoide	1	0	2
Colonic ADK	3	0	0
Bronchopulmonary cancer	2	0	0
Primary glial tumor	1	0	0

ADK of the neck	0	0	1
Carcinoma of the lower esophagus	1	0	0
ADKcharnerecto-sigmoidal	1	0	0
Hepatic cholangiocarcinoma	1	0	0
UCNT	1	0	0
ADK: adenocarcinoma; EC: squamous cell carcinoma; UCNT: undifferentiated carcinoma of nasopharyngeal type			

The patients, for whom the diagnosis of NPCI was retained, all had a length-dependent axonal damage affecting mainly the sural nerve at the level of its sensitive amplitude (Table V).

Table V: Neuropathic damage according to the sensitive amplitude of the sural nerve

Sensory amplitude of the sural nerve	*G1 Platinum derivatives*	*G2 Taxanes*	*G3 low toxicity*	*G4 Witnesses*
	N=17	*N= 6*	*N= 6*	*N=8*
≥20 μV	12	2	6	8
<20 μV	5	4	0	0

Comparing the 3 chemotherapy groups with a control group, there was a significant difference between the 4 groups in the sensitive amplitude of the sural nerve and its sensitive nerve conduction velocity, and the sensitive amplitude of the musculocutaneous nerve.

Table VI: *Comparison of parameters of sensitive nerve conduction in the lower limbs*

	G1Derivatives of platinum N=34 (17)	G2 Taxanes N= 12 (6)	G3 Witnesses N= 12 (6)	G4 LB L5 N=16 (8)	Kruskall-Wallis test p=
ASSural (µV)	N=33 21,56 ± 8,43* IC95%[18.7; 25]	N=12 16,13 ± 8,14* IC95%[11.2; 22.2]	N= 12 31,66 ± 8,41* IC95%[26.8; 39.5]	N=16 27,81 ±7,7* IC95%[23.7; 31.9]	0,000**
VCS Sural (m/s)	N=33 49,04 ± 7,47* IC95%[46.4; 52.3]	N=12 43,55 ± 7,11* IC95%[39.6; 48.9]	N=12 50,88 ± 7,48* IC95%[47; 57.7]	N=16 52,93± 7,64* IC95%[48.8; 57]	0,014**
ASM SC (µV)	N=34 22,39 ± 9,6* IC95%[18.5; 25.4]	N=12 12,79 ± 5,02* IC95%[9.8; 16.6]	N=11 23,08 ± 8,03* IC95%[18.6; 30.7]	N=16 27,6± 10,82* IC95%[21.8; 33.3]	0,001**
VCS MSC (m/s)	N=34 52,24 ± 7,24* IC95%[49.6; 55.2]	N= 11 49,37 ± 9,27* IC95%[43.1; 55.6]	N=9 50,52 ± 5,6* IC95%[46.2; 54.8]	N=16 52,05± 5,79* IC95%[48.9; 55.1]	0,535

*AS: sensory amplitude; MSC: musculocutaneous nerve; SVC: sensory conduction velocity; *mean ± standard deviation; ** $p<0,05$*

According to the post-hoc test, the sensitive amplitude of the sural nerve is significantly more diminished for G2 than for G3 ($p=0.011$) and for G4 (p=0.001). It is also more decreased for G1 compared to G3 ($p=0.022$). The sensitive conduction velocity of the sural nerve was significantly more diminished in G2 than in G4 ($p=0.012$). The sensitive amplitude of the musculocutaneous nerve was significantly more diminished for G2 compared to G1 ($p=0.006$), for G2 compared tG3 ($p=0.048$) and for G2 compared to G4 ($p=0.001$). The motor amplitude of the SPE nerve was significantly more decreased for G2 compared to G4 ($p=0.035$). The motor amplitude of the SPI nerve is significantly more decreased for G2 compared to G4 ($p=0.015$), G1 compared to G4 ($p=0.001$) and G3 compared to G4 ($p=0.02$)

Table VII: *Comparison of motor nerve conduction parameters in the lower limbs*

	G1 Platinum derivatives N=34 (17)	G2 Taxanes N= 12 (6)	G3 a low N= 12 (6)	G4 control N=16 (8)	Kruskall-wallis test p=	from
AMSPE (µV)	N= 32	N= 12	N=12	N=16		
	4,88 ± 2,38*	3,84 ± 1,88*	4,94 ± 1,32*	6,08±1,69*	0,05	
	CI95%[4.3; 6]	IC95%[2.7; 5.2]	IC95%[4.1; 5.7]	IC95%[5.1; 6.9]		
VCM SPE (m/s)	N=29	N=12	N=12	N=16		
	44,99 ± 7,76*	45,74 ± 3,43*	44,97 ± 4,29*	48,46± 4,92*	0,264	
	IC95%[42; 47.9]	IC95%[43,2 ;48]	IC95%[41.7 ;48.3]	IC95%[45.8; 51]		
AMSPI (µV)	N= 32	N= 12	N= 12	N=16		
	6,79 ± 1,98*	7 ± 2,96*	6,96 ± 1,85*	10,07± 2,55*	0,001	
	IC95%[6.1; 7.6]	IC95%[5; 9.1]	IC95%[5.9; 8.7]	IC95%[8.7; 11.4]		

*AM: motor amplitude; EPS: lateral popliteal sciatica; IPS: medial popliteal sciatica (medial tibial nerve); MVC: motor conduction velocity; *mean ± standard deviation*

When looking for a cut-off value for the cures whatever the chemotherapy (taxanes or DP), the 6ème cure appeared to be this value showing a significantly decreased value for the sural nerve amplitude for less than 6 cures with a mean of 13.55±9.91 µV (N=31) compared to a number of cures from 6 with a mean of 22.94±9.83 µV (N=8) with $p=0.021$

Discussion

This is a particularly revealing study of the magnitude of the neurotoxic effect of Taxanes compared to PDs. Despite the fact that the NPCI of PDs is the best known, however, for the same cumulative dose, it would appear that Taxanes would more rapidly produce a neuropathy diagnosed by nerve conduction studies. NPCI secondary to PD appears to occur at higher cumulative doses (43). All our patients were referred for the appearance of paresthesias of the limbs classifying the patients in the first three clinical grades, whatever the scale used (Table (39)). However, not all of them were diagnosed with polyneuropathy. These subjective symptoms would probably be secondary to other causes, particularly small fiber involvement, which would not be explored by the ENMG (44).

This study, being retrospective, does not lack bias. Indeed, the patients did not have an ENMG before the start of chemotherapy, which could give us information on the state of their nerves before and after treatment, thus allowing us to have intra-patient standards and the degree of nerve damage secondary to the treatment itself (45). Patients could not be selected on the basis of their neoplastic pathology in order to eliminate any selection bias by eliminating any patient with a pathology inducing polyneuropathy. This could lead to a confounding bias, the degree of impact of the disease itself in generating neuropathy. There is an information bias, in that there is a lack of information about the cumulative doses of chemotherapy and the onset of symptoms. Patients could not be followed according to their cumulative dose of treatment, which could have been indicative of the key dose causing NPCI (45). The 1[er] chemotherapy group was treated with Platinum Derivatives which are platinum-based chemotherapy drugs include cisplatin, carboplatin and oxaliplatin (43). Others are used in some countries including nedaplatin (Japan), heptaplatin (South Korea), and lobaplatin (China) (43). Cisplatin is a cytotoxic anti-cancer drug used since 1972 (46). It is a heavy metal complex with a central platinum atom. It is indicated for ovarian, testicular, endometrial, small-cell bronchial, and solid tumors in children. It acts by inhibiting DNA synthesis through the formation of intra- and inter-strand chromosomal bonds (46). Mitochondrial destruction is also thought to play a role in the genesis of neuropathy (43). It usually causes a large-fiber sensory polyneuropathy with deficits in vibration and proprioception leading to ataxia (43). There is also lesser small fiber involvement (43). Despite the small fiber loss, pain is marked in most forms of NPCI; autonomic symptoms are also less frequent; and muscle weakness is atypical in part because of minimal drug access to motor neurons protected by the blood-brain barrier (43). The same impairment is reportedly described for oxaliplatin (43). The risk of developing neuropathy increases at doses exceeding 75 mg/m2 for cisplatin and at cumulative doses exceeding 800 mg/m2 for oxaliplatin (43). The 2ème chemotherapy group was treated with Taxanes drugs which are a class of anticancer agents, designed to treat a variety of cancers: ovarian, breast, non-small cell lung and prostate (43). Paclitaxel and docetaxel represent this drug class. Docetaxel is a semi-synthetic molecule, prepared from a precursor extracted from the needles of the European yew tree, *Taxus baccata*. Paclitaxel (Taxol) is derived from the bark of the Pacific yew, *Taxus brevifolia*, which is thus a readily renewable source (46). Carbazitaxel was introduced in 2010 (43). This drug class can cause a predominantly sensory neuropathy, a few days after the 1ère dose. This neuropathy is cumulative and dose-dependent, and symptoms typically improve within a few days and recur after each treatment cycle; approximately all patients develop symptoms after the 3ème cycle. Initial complaints include numbness and pain, and neuropathy may involve both small- and large-diameter sensory fibers, autonomic nerves, and sometimes cranial nerves; motor involvement is typically minimal only if the dose is higher than conventional (43). The therapeutic action of Taxanes appears to be an interruption of microtubule function, leading to accumulation, assembly and thus altering their axonal transport and preventing their depolymerization by binding to the β-subunit (46). These microtubules will aggregate in an increased manner, stabilize and regroup in the axons thus stiffening the sensory neurons. These microtubules are then stable enough to prevent further mitosis and thus lead to the death of the cancer cell (46). There is also a role for the release of substance P in the dorsal surface layers of the spinal cord and a disruption of nuclear mRNA transport (43). Despite the fact that the number of patients used in G2 is small and that almost half of them have just had their 1ère treatment at the time of their chemotherapy and ENMG, the degree of impact of their treatment on their sensory amplitudes in the lower limbs can be seen compared with the other groups (45). Indeed, this is consistent with the results of other studies, where Taxanes are incriminated as early as 1ère administration (4, 6, 43). Moreover, it is comforting to know that the neoplastic pathologies of which these patients are affected (breast carcinoma and ovarian adenocarcinoma) are rarely associated with paraneoplastic neuropathies (42). However, the low level of motor impairment secondary to the 2 drug classes is clearly noticeable, but more apparent for Taxanes. Indeed, some studies report an axonopathy effect exerted on the cells of the anterior horn of the spinal cord by Taxanes, which would be at the origin of an apparent motor impairment for these molecules (47, 48). As for the sensory impairment, it would be in line with the data in the literature, where an action is described which appears on the dorsal surface of the spinal cord and could in this case give rise to a sensory neuronopathy (41). However, this diagnosis remains difficult on a practical level, particularly when one is faced with distal symmetrical attacks that are particularly predominant in the lower limbs, as is the case in our study (41, 49). A study in animals (mice) showed that those treated with Taxanes and vincristine developed distal axonal sensory neuropathy more rapidly than those treated with cisplatin and bortezomib (19). The same study showed, by histological sections, that the sciatic nerve of mice had a significant reduction in myelinated fibers when treated with cisplatin (19).

In an in-vitro study in rat dorsal root ganglia, it was found that at concentrations of cisplatin and oxaliplatin and paclitaxel lower than

those required for neurotoxicity, cytotoxicity was induced and myelin basic protein expression was reduced (49). These same drugs disrupted myelin formation in dorsal ganglia Schwann cells without affecting the nerve axon. Cisplatin and oxaliplatin were reported to cause mitochondrial dysfunction in cultured Schwann cells. This is in contrast to paclitaxel, which caused Schwann cells to differentiate into an immature state, characterized by increased expression of p75 and galectin-3 (49). This damage would be important in the development of CINP in conjunction with direct damage to peripheral neurons (49). However, these myelin damages described are not reflected by the nerve conduction performed in our patients where the slowing of conduction velocities would reflect more the impact of the axonal damage than the demyelination itself. However, this could explain the onset of neuropathy after less than 6 courses of treatment for both DP and Taxanes, suggesting an early mechanism of action independent of the cumulative dose. In the long term, it appears that Taxane-induced neuropathy has a good prognosis
(50) and may even be improved by exercise (51).

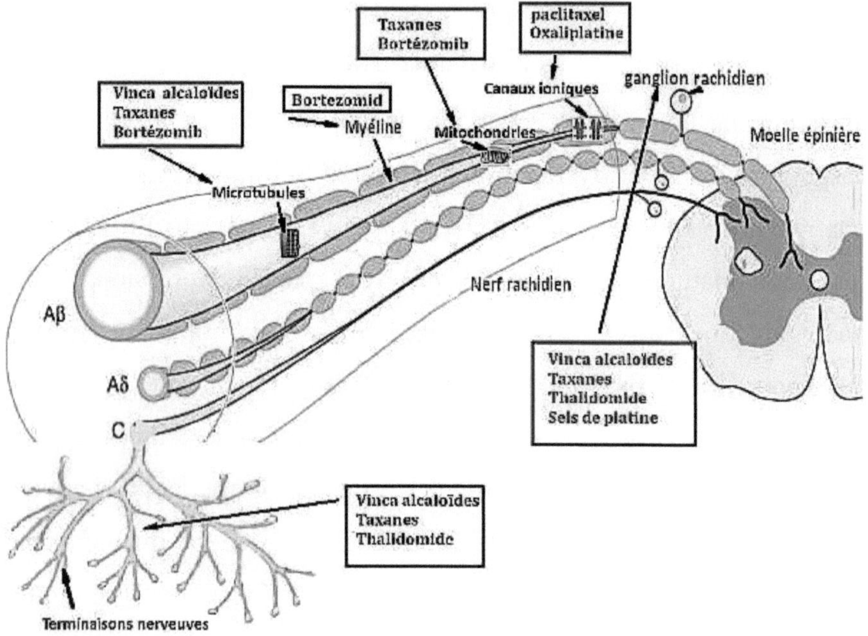

Figure 1: The main neurotoxic effects of chemotherapies according to the contribution of experimental models (reference: https://meridiens.org/meridienjmstephf/neuropathies-peripheriques-induites-par-la-chemotherapy-mechanisms-action-of-lacupuncture-in-peripheral-and-central-sensitization/)

Conclusion

The mechanism of neuropathy induction is not the same for the two molecules, but it seems that the mechanism of Taxanes is more direct and rapid. It would be interesting to carry out other prospective studies highlighting the difference in the neurotoxicity of each chemotherapeutic treatment and thus allowing the clinical oncologist to be cautious at each treatment cycle and probably to plan a stop of the treatment and a switch to another molecule before the onset of NPCI, which could be disabling and embarrassing for the patient

References

1. Lagueny A, Vital A. Toxic neuropathies. Elsevier Masson SAS. 2008;Neurology.
2. Chaudhry V, Rowinsky EK, Sartorius SE, Donehower RC, Cornblath DR. Peripheral neuropathy from taxol and cisplatin combination chemotherapy: clinical and electrophysiological studies. Annals of neurology. 1994;35(3):304-11.
3. Lebrun C, Frenay M, Lanteri-Minet M. [Neurologic complications of chemotherapy]. La Revue de medecine interne. 1999;20(10):902-11.
4. Lebrun C, Frenay M. [Neurologic side effects of cytotoxic drugs]. La Revue de medecine interne. 2010;31(4):295-304.
5. Huang H-W, Wu P-Y, Su P-F, Li C-I, Yeh Y-M, Lin P-C, et al. A Simplified Diagnostic Classification Scheme of Chemotherapy-Induced Peripheral Neuropathy. Disease Markers. 2020;2020:3402108.
6. Brewer JR, Morrison G, Dolan ME, Fleming GF. Chemotherapy-induced peripheral neuropathy: Current status and progress. Gynecologic oncology. 2016;140(1):176-83.
7. Ewertz M, Qvortrup C, Eckhoff L. Chemotherapy-induced peripheral neuropathy in patients treated with taxanes and platinum derivatives. Acta oncologica (Stockholm, Sweden). 2015;54(5):587-91.
8. Misra UK, Kalita J, Nair PP. Diagnostic approach to peripheral neuropathy. Annals of Indian Academy of Neurology. 2008;11(2):89-97.
9. Argyriou AA, Polychronopoulos P, Iconomou G, Koutras A, Kalofonos HP, Chroni E. Paclitaxel plus carboplatin-induced peripheral neuropathy. A prospective clinical and electrophysiological study in patients suffering from solid malignancies. Journal of neurology. 2005;252(12):1459-64.
10. Novello BJ, Pobre T. Electrodiagnostic Evaluation Of Peripheral Neuropathy. StatPearls. Treasure Island, FL: StatPearls Publishing.

Copyright © 2021, StatPearls Publishing LLC; 2021.
11. Grisold W, Cavaletti G, Windebank AJ. Peripheral neuropathies from chemotherapeutics and targeted agents: diagnosis, treatment, and prevention. Neuro-oncology. 2012;14 Suppl 4(Suppl 4):iv45-54.
12. Magistris HGAKATMR. Sensory neuropathies. Swiss medical journal. 2007 MAY 9. 2007.
13. Menzin AW, King SA, Aikins JK, Mikuta JJ, Rubin SC. Taxol (paclitaxel) was approved by FDA for the treatment of patients with recurrent ovarian cancer. Gynecologic oncology. 1994;54(1):103.

14. Velasco R, Bruna J. Taxane-Induced Peripheral Neurotoxicity. Toxics. 2015;3(2):152-69.
15. Tamburin S, Park SB, Alberti P, Demichelis C, Schenone A, Argyriou AA. Taxane and epothilone-induced peripheral neurotoxicity: From pathogenesis to treatment. Journal of the peripheral nervous system: JPNS. 2019;24 Suppl 2:S40-s51.
16. Verweij J, Clavel M, Chevalier B. Paclitaxel (Taxol) and docetaxel (Taxotere): not simply two of a kind. Annals of oncology : official journal of the European Society for Medical Oncology. 1994;5(6):495-505.
17. Stubblefield MD, Burstein HJ, Burton AW, Custodio CM, Deng GE, Ho M, et al. NCCN task force report: management of neuropathy in cancer. Journal of the National Comprehensive Cancer Network: JNCCN. 2009;7 Suppl 5:S1- S26; quiz S7-8.
18. Song SJ, Min J, Suh SY, Jung SH, Hahn HJ, Im SA, et al. Incidence of taxane-induced peripheral neuropathy receiving treatment and prescription patterns in patients with breast cancer. Supportive care in cancer: official journal of the Multinational Association of Supportive Care in Cancer. 2017;25(7):2241-8.
19. Boehmerle W, Huehnchen P, Peruzzaro S, Balkaya M, Endres M. Electrophysiological, behavioral and histological characterization of paclitaxel, cisplatin, vincristine and bortezomib-induced neuropathy in C57Bl/6 mice. Scientific reports. 2014;4:6370.
20. Nirschl JJ, Ghiretti AE, Holzbaur ELF. The impact of cytoskeletal organization on the local regulation of neuronal transport. Nature reviews Neuroscience. 2017;18(10):585-97.
21. Gornstein E, Schwarz TL. The paradox of paclitaxel neurotoxicity: Mechanisms and unanswered questions. Neuropharmacology. 2014;76 Pt A:175-83.
22. Cook BM, Wozniak KM, Proctor DA, Bromberg RB, Wu Y, Slusher BS, et al. Differential Morphological and Biochemical Recovery from Chemotherapy-Induced Peripheral Neuropathy Following Paclitaxel, Ixabepilone, or Eribulin Treatment in Mouse Sciatic Nerves. Neurotoxicity research. 2018;34(3):677-92.
23. Staff NP, Grisold A, Grisold W, Windebank AJ. Chemotherapy-induced peripheral neuropathy: A current review. Annals of neurology. 2017;81(6):772- 81.

24. Was H, Borkowska A, Bagues A, Tu L, Liu JYH, Lu Z, et al.

Mechanisms of Chemotherapy-Induced Neurotoxicity. 2022;13.
25. Fischer JaG, C.R. Analogue-Based Drug Discovery. John Wiley & Sons, Hoboken. 2006:504.
26. Johnstone TC, Suntharalingam K, Lippard SJ. The Next Generation of Platinum Drugs: Targeted Pt(II) Agents, Nanoparticle Delivery, and Pt(IV) Prodrugs. Chemical reviews. 2016;116(5):3436-86.
27. Rabik CA, Dolan ME. Molecular mechanisms of resistance and toxicity associated with platinating agents. Cancer treatment reviews. 2007;33(1):9-23.
28. Dzagnidze A, Katsarava Z, Makhalova J, Liedert B, Yoon MS, Kaube H, et al. Repair capacity for platinum-DNA adducts determines the severity of cisplatin-induced peripheral neuropathy. The Journal of neuroscience : the official journal of the Society for Neuroscience. 2007;27(35):9451-7.
29. Podratz JL, Staff NP, Froemel D, Wallner A, Wabnig F, Bieber AJ, et al. Drosophila melanogaster: a new model to study cisplatin-induced neurotoxicity. Neurobiology of disease. 2011;43(2):330-7.
30. Wang JT, Medress ZA, Barres BA. Axon degeneration: molecular mechanisms of a self-destruction pathway. The Journal of cell biology. 2012;196(1):7-18.
31. Shen S, Lim G, You Z, Ding W, Huang P, Ran C, et al. Gut microbiota is critical for the induction of chemotherapy-induced pain. Nature neuroscience. 2017;20(9):1213-6.
32. BORIES-AZEAU L. Severe sensorimotor neuropathy after cisplatin therapy. 1985.
33. Boogerd W, ten Bokkel Huinink WW, Dalesio O, Hoppenbrouwers WJ, van der Sande JJ. Cisplatin induced neuropathy: central, peripheral and autonomic nerve involvement. Journal of neuro-oncology. 1990;9(3):255-63.
34. Canetta R, Rozencweig M, Carter SK. Carboplatin: the clinical spectrum to date. Cancer treatment reviews. 1985;12 Suppl A:125-36.
35. Grothey A. Clinical management of oxaliplatin-associated neurotoxicity. Clinical colorectal cancer. 2005;5 Suppl 1:S38-46.
36. Omran M, Belcher EK, Mohile NA, Kesler SR, Janelsins MC, Hohmann AG, et al. Review of the Role of the Brain in Chemotherapy-Induced Peripheral Neuropathy. Frontiers in molecular biosciences. 2021;8:693133.
37. Zajączkowska R, Kocot-Kępska M, Leppert W, Wrzosek A, Mika J, Wordliczek J. Mechanisms of Chemotherapy-Induced Peripheral Neuropathy. International journal of molecular sciences. 2019;20(6).
38. https://www.cen-neurologie.fr/deuxieme-cycle/deficit-neurologique-

recent [
39. Bridges CM, Smith EM. What about Alice? Peripheral neuropathy from taxane-containing treatment for advanced nonsmall cell lung cancer. Supportive care in cancer: official journal of the Multinational Association of Supportive Care in Cancer. 2014;22(9):2581-92.
40. Argyriou AA, Kyritsis AP, Makatsoris T, Kalofonos HP. Chemotherapy-induced peripheral neuropathy in adults: a comprehensive update of the literature. Cancer management and research. 2014;6:135-47.
41. CAMDESSANCHE JP. Acquired sensory neuropathies: diagnoses you must not miss; Sensory neuropathies: diagnoses you mustn't miss. The Neurologist's Letter. 2012;16:226-30.
42. Antoine JC, Camdessanché JP. Paraneoplastic neuropathies. Current opinion in neurology. 2017;30(5):513-20.
43. Cioroiu C, Weimer LH. Update on Chemotherapy-Induced Peripheral Neuropathy. Current neurology and neuroscience reports. 2017;17(6):47.
44. Ginsberg L. Acute and chronic neuropathies. Medicine (Abingdon, England: UK ed). 2020;48(9):612-8.
45. Augusto C, Pietro M, Cinzia M, Sergio C, Sara C, Luca G, et al. Peripheral neuropathy due to paclitaxel: study of the temporal relationships between the therapeutic schedule and the clinical quantitative score (QST) and comparison with neurophysiological findings. Journal of neuro-oncology. 2008;86(1):89-99.
46. P Bouche JL, JM Vallat. Peripheral neuropathies. Multiple polyneuropathies and mononeuropathies. jle.com ed2003. 404 p.
47. Freilich RJ, Balmaceda C, Seidman AD, Rubin M, DeAngelis LM. Motor neuropathy due to docetaxel and paclitaxel. Neurology. 1996;47(1):115-8.
48. Molassiotis A, Cheng HL, Lopez V, Au JSK, Chan A, Bandla A, et al. Are we mis-estimating chemotherapy-induced peripheral neuropathy? Analysis of assessment methodologies from a prospective, multinational, longitudinal cohort study of patients receiving neurotoxic chemotherapy. BMC cancer. 2019;19(1):132.
49. Imai S, Koyanagi M, Azimi Z, Nakazato Y, Matsumoto M, Ogihara T, et al. Taxanes and platinum derivatives impair Schwann cells via distinct mechanisms. Scientific reports. 2017;7(1):5947.
50. Osmani K, Vignes S, Aissi M, Wade F, Milani P, Lévy BI, et al. Taxane- induced peripheral neuropathy has good long-term prognosis: a 1- to

13-year evaluation. Journal of neurology. 2012;259(9):1936-43.
51. Bland KA, Kirkham AA, Bovard J, Shenkier T, Zucker D, McKenzie DC, et al. Effect of Exercise on Taxane Chemotherapy-Induced Peripheral Neuropathy in Women With Breast Cancer: A Randomized Controlled Trial. Clinical breast cancer. 2019;19(6):411-22.

Annexes

Appendix: Chemotherapy-induced neuropathy and clinical symptoms (24)

Drug	Type of neuropathy	Clinical symptoms
Cisplatin/oxaliplatin	Pure sensory	Paresthesia Dysesthesia Neuropathic pain in a stocking-and-glove distribution
Acute oxaliplatin		Paresthesia Muscle tightness Cramps
Paclitaxel	Mixed sensory—motor	Paresthesia Hypoesthesia Neuropathic pain in a stocking-and-glove distribution Myalgia, myopathy
Vincristine	Mixed sensory-motor and autonomic	Paresthesia Hypoesthesia Neuropathic pain in a stocking-and-glove distribution Muscle cramps Mild distal weakness Enteric neuropathy Autonomic dysfunctions
Bortezomib and thalidomide	Sensory-motor	Neuropathic pain Hypoesthesia Paresthesia in distal extremities of limbs Muscle cramps
Bortezomib	Sensory-motor (rare) and autonomic	Paresthesia Painful sensory neuropathy in distal extremities of limbs

Table 1. Classification of definite paraneoplastic neuropathies

Neuropathy	Cancer	Reported case number	Abs and other biomarkers	Other criteria for definite paraneoplastic	Comments
Neuronopathies					
Sensory neuronopathy	SCLC 80% – HL and other carcinoma	>500	Hu, CV2/CRMP5, other onconeural		One case with Ma2 Abs and NHL
lower motor neuron disease	SCLC-HL-carcinoma	<20 cases	Hu with SCLC only	Some improved with tumor treatment	Rare cases Ma2 Abs
Mixed sensory and motor	SCLC-70%	>200	Hu		According to presentation, may be confused with different forms of axonal sensory motor neuropathy
Autonomic neuropathy	SCLC 70% – HL and other carcinoma	SCLC<200 – other <10	Hu, (ganglionic AChR)	Some with HL improved with immunotherapy	Frequently associated with SSN and anti-Hu Abs
Sensory-motor neuropathies without gammopathy					
Axonal	Carcinoma and HL	Rare	Usually none	Some improved with tumor treatment	Rare cases with Yo or Ma2 Abs
Axonal and demyelinating	SCLC and thymoma	<50 with CV2/ CRMP5 AB	CV2/CRMP5		Frequently associated with CNS involvement with CV2/CRMP5 Abs
Demyalinating (CIDP)	Carcinoma and NHL	<50	Rarely CV2/CRMP5	Some improved with tumor treatment	With NHL, neurolymphomatosis is the differential diagnosis
vasculitic neuropathy	SCLC, NHL, and other carcinoma	<50	Rarely Hu	Some improved with tumor treatment	
Sensory-motor neuropathies with gammopathy					
Axonal sensory and painful	AL amyloidosis and myeloma	>500	free light chains		multisystemic organ involvement
Démyelinating	Waldenströem	>500	anti-MAG IgM k		mostly sensory and distal, tremor
	NHL	<10	antiganglioside IgM		CANOMAD or motor neuropathy according to Abs activity
	Osteosclerotic myeloma and plasmocytoma (POEMS)	>400	IgG I VEGF		multisystemic organ involvement
Vasculitic neuropathy	type I cryoglobulinemia lymphopathy	>200	Cryoglobulin and low complement level		Mostly sensory and multisystemic organ involvement
Neuromyotonia	Thymoma (SCLC and NHL) 30%	<100	Caspr2 and Netrin 1 receptor		Insomnia, delirium with Morvan syndrome. Myasthenia gravis frequent

Abs, antibodies; HL, Hodgkin's lymphoma; NHL, non-Hodgkin's lymphoma; POEMS polyneuropathy-organomegaly-endocrinopathy-M component-skin changes; SCLC, small cell lung cancer; VEGF, vascular endothelial growth factor.

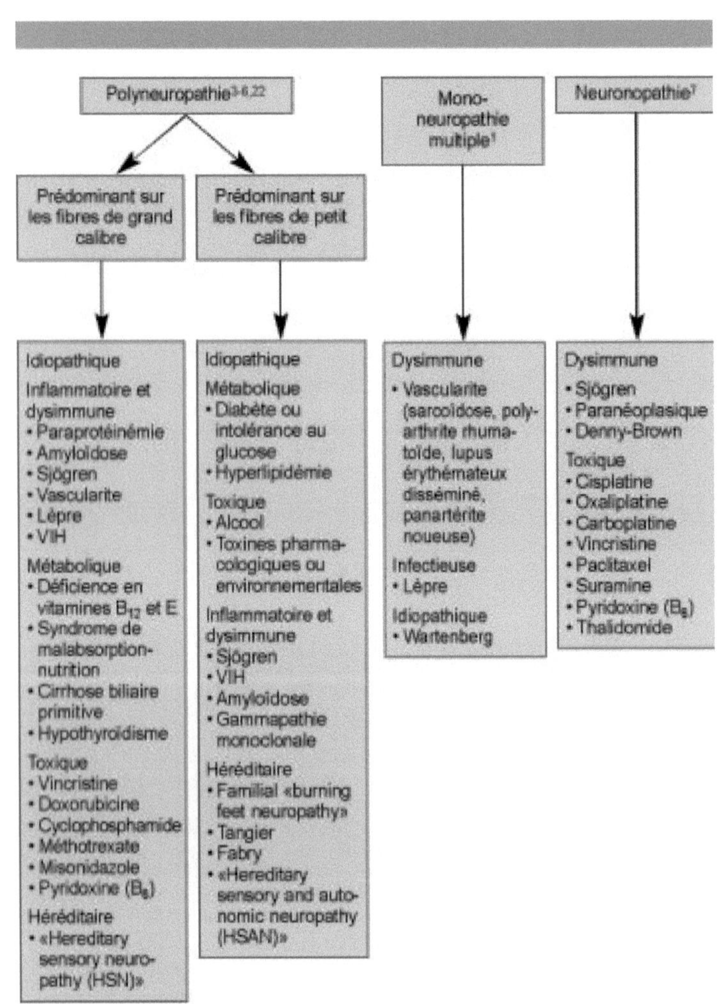

Figure 1. Causes des neuropathies sensitives

Photos: method of acquisition of nerve conduction in the lower limbs

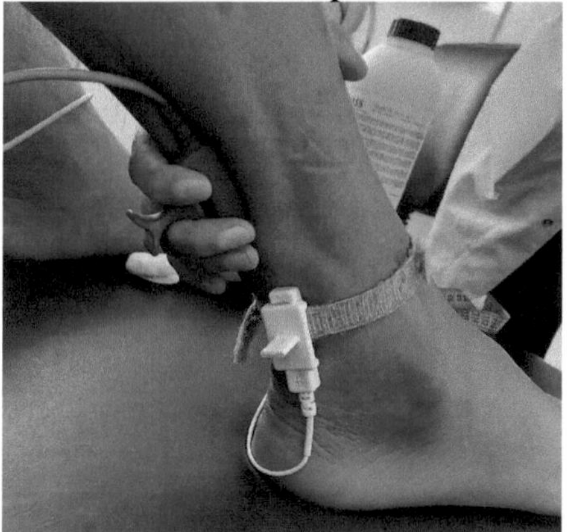

Photo 1 : Signal acquisition method for the sural nerve

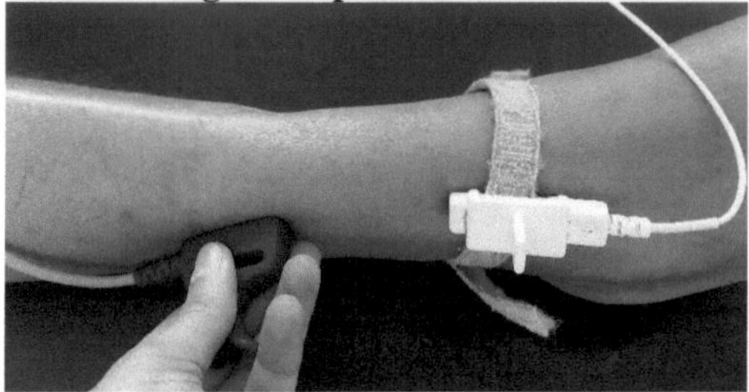

Photo 2: Signal acquisition method for the musculocutaneous nerve

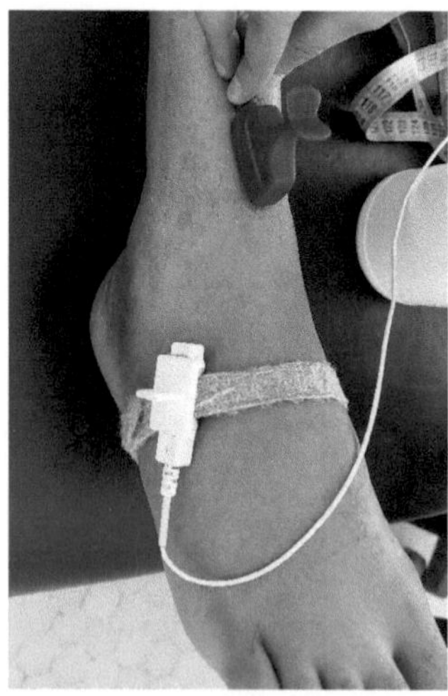

Photo 3: Signal acquisition method for the SPE nerve with distal stimulation (ankle)

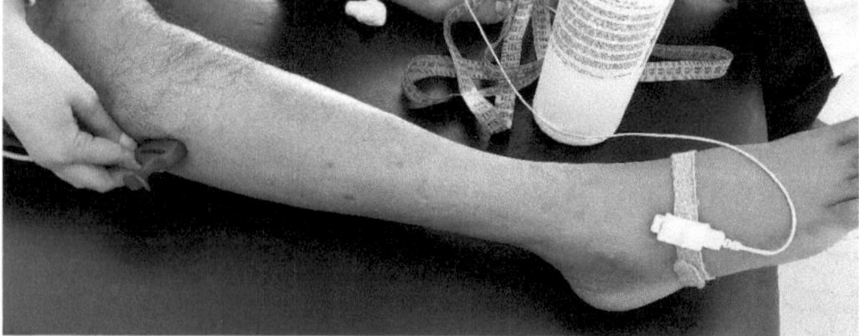

Photo 4: Signal acquisition method for the SPE nerve with proximal stimulation (under the head of the fibula)

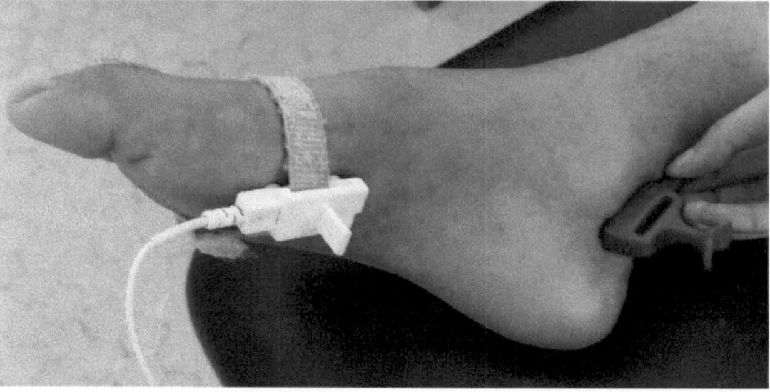

Photo 5: Signal acquisition method for the SPI nerve with distal stimulation (ankle in retro-malleolar)

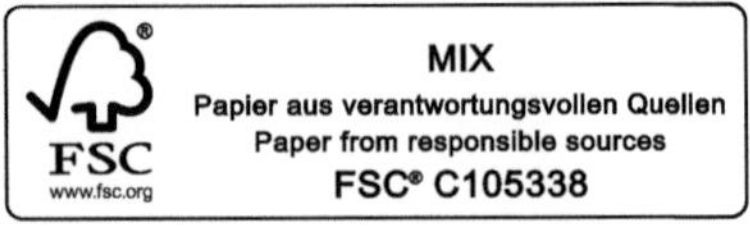

Printed by Books on Demand GmbH, Norderstedt / Germany